8225

Parents

DATE DUE

MAR 21			

D0557199

Early Flight

Healing
Hope for Parents
of the Stillborn,
Miscarried or Aborted

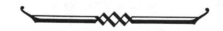

by Jack Hayford

EARLY FLIGHT: Healing Hope for Parents of the Stillborn,
Miscarried or Aborted
International Standard Book Number: 0-916847-06-3
Library of Congress Catalog Card Number: 86-82456

 LIVING WAY MINISTRIES

Copyright ©1986 Jack W. Hayford
Published by Living Way Ministries
Van Nuys, CA 91405-2499

Table of Contents

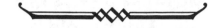

" . . . The fundamental assignment Jesus gave is to go into the world with *good* news for broken people."

Introduction

Abortion is not only a tough topic but an incredibly delicate one. And it's a tragedy.

But my object in these pages is not to elaborate that tragedy or underscore the facts of human failure. Rather, I seek to offer hope, comfort and direction for the future.

That's the focus, and the subject I deal with here is broader than abortion. I'm concerned with the death of any child who misses life's potential because of *either* miscarriage, stillbirth or abortion. And I'm concerned about the pain, the aftermath of emotion felt by a woman, a couple or a family who have lost a child.

Sadly, "hope" is a word and a concept these people seldom encounter.

Most mothers who choose abortion are *not* indifferent to the child within. As misguided as their decisions may be — promoted and legalized by a society temporarily numbed to the truest values of human life — women consenting to an abortion have feelings. And our eyes need to be opened to see Jesus Himself reaching in tenderness to those in the aftermath of abortion. I *must* care — *we* must — even though their pain is the result of their own decision.

However often the Church may be called to resensitize the conscience of society, at the same time we must be careful to show understanding, compassion and tenderness. Indignation and demonstration may be provoked, but the fundamental assignment Jesus gave is to go into the world with *good* news for broken people.

And to offer hope.

So, dear reader, I ask you to patiently hear those who are broken. Perhaps you, like I, have had to wrestle against bitterness or self-righteousness; condemnation rising from your own emotions, and permeating your attitude toward others.

I did. And though I hated to admit it, I found those very things in my own heart. I was not only angry that lives were being taken, but I felt superior. And that was the hateful blindness I had to deal with: the cocksureness of my self-righteous opinon. In that state I couldn't even begin to gain perspective on the fear, pain, hurt, agony and embarrassment of so many who needed something else from me. Society has so liberalized abortion that the uninformed and uncounselled readily give in, until in the aftermath of the experience, the living victims bend beneath another burden — the burden of questions.

"What have I done?"
"Who might the child have become?"
"Was I right? Wrong? Can I never forget?"
"What would have happened if I hadn't?"

As a pastor — a shepherd of souls — I was encountering situations that gave me an inside look at the brutal reality of this social tragedy. I was meeting people in the aftermath; walking through the emotional carnage after abortion — some believing they were wrong, others uncertain. Those experiences didn't change my convictions about the wrongness of abortion, but they cured my soul of the wrongness of my superficial point of view. I began to see a place where life, light and love are desperately needed — a place in our world where truth not only can shine like a beacon light discerning between good and evil, but where that same truth can also shed the light of healing, freedom, warmth and hope-fullness.

So, I began to search God's Word for a sound basis for my case. I wasn't seeking to build a case against human failure, as surely as that might be proven, but I wanted to find the Bible's offer of a case for hope in the midst of this particular sin's aftermath. I wanted to find truth to heal and to give comfort in the midst of the pain following the amputation of a life from its present potential. And in doing this, I encountered another group of sufferers: People who had planned, prepared and prayed for a child. But their baby was stillborn — dead on arrival. And what about the thousands whose newborn babes lived so short a life as to have hardly, truly arrived; babies who died a few hours, days or weeks after birth? Together, parents of the stillborn and of the newly born who die, form a distinct group: people who had a baby they never got to keep.

And there is yet a third group of the disappointed: Hosts of women who had longed for a child; but two, three — four or maybe five — months into their pregnancy something went awry and they miscarried. Now there's a new set of questions:

"Was it an act of God, somehow penalizing me for an action long-past?"

"Did I do something wrong? Could it be I'm unworthy . . . a failure?"

"Should I allow myself to expect — to hope again?"

And these questions are being asked by larger numbers than I would have guessed — the parents of the stillborn, the miscarrying mother, and the maternal victim of abortion — *parents of a child* potentially designed for a lifetime of fulfillment and purpose. In the Creator's finest plan these children were not intended for the disease, death or destruction that took their lives. But they died. Like a rescheduled airplane suddenly departing ahead of time, these took an "early flight." Before we ever could know them . . . their possibilities . . . their presence and purpose, they were gone. Whether their hastened departure was forced through accident, neglect or abuse of the fetus — whether through disease, deformity or simple malfunction — suddenly they departed.

And it is to those who remain at the airport of the present, with tears, pain, bitterness or questions, that I dedicate these moments in God's Word; truth which I hold forth with hope. And at the same moment, by God's Spirit, I hold yet another hope.

I hope that among those of us who may have never known such pain, failure or grief, an enlargement of heart may occur. May His Spirit speaking His Word create a new space within *all* of us, making a place where we can host with understanding and compassion all those we know or will meet, who have been "left at the gate" so to speak — standing at the terminal end of things following a little one's early flight from this life's promise. There is hope to find and to share, for the "terminal" on our side doesn't have a view of the destination on theirs.

So, come with me to the fountain of truth — to God's Word, where eternal wisdom, reconciling righteousness and healing hope abound. Let's find out what we can about God's answers to one of the most frequently experienced traumas in our present society; the pain following an "early flight."

"And the Lord God formed man of the dust of the ground and breathed into his nostrils the breath of life, and man became a living being."

(Genesis 2:7)

Chapter 1

The Gift of *Lives*

I run a very real risk in examining the subject of abortion as I intend to. It is entirely possible that someone may falsely interpret my seeking to offer comfort, concluding on their part that correction is needed instead. But my quest in the Scriptures is not prompted by a casual attitude toward the fact that fetuses are being killed. Instead, I want to answer questions:

    . . . questions that have sometimes been asked too late;

    . . . questions that have hardly found expression because the inquirer stifled them within, before the heart could complete their phrasing.

"You shouldn't have . . . ," "God knows and cares. . . ." Neither accusations nor platitudes, no matter how graciously intended, no matter how justified their legal or theological grounds, can ever offer soul-satisfying answers. And they will never bring real hope or comfort.

So where shall we start in providing healing truth; in offering real life where death has come by means of a child's early flight?

Perhaps the best place is to first answer this question: "Was this yet unborn child, in the fullest sense of the word, *actually* a human being?" That question must be settled with confidence and personal certainty. God's answer gives rise to an amazing basis for hope — an expectancy never before anticipated as possible. So let's discover what the Creator Himself has to say on the subject, and turn to the Word of God — the Scriptures, the Holy Bible.

Our first objective is to establish a biblical basis for the prenatal existence of the human soul. Is a person a person *before* they are born?

Here is the crux of the issue, for if we are only dealing with chemistry or tissue, in examining the nature of the fetus or the stillborn, there is little at stake. But in most of us an inner monitor signals that there *is* something more involved here than mere chemical combinations or complex structures of tissues. Could it be that God has given a conclusive and confirming witness in His Word, to companion with that internal sense most everyone shares — that the life of an embryo is eternal?

Without surrendering to either mystery or superstition, we can assertively say, "Yes!" The life of the child in the womb *is* eternal. But please be clear on this:This is a statement born from far more than either religious opinion or occult dogma.

The religionist may trumpet the *reality* of, and therefore the sanctity of, life in the womb. But so often these assertions lead to the levelling of accusations. The reincarnationist proposes that all human life is merely the recycling of personalities in new bodies, with hopes on ever-improving one's lot in life with each recycling experience. Whatever the wish, hope or pretended logic of such a proposition, honesty requires that we immediately dispense with those notions. God's Word abolishes the phantom philosophies of reincarnation. According to the final revelation of the Bible, life is a one-time proposition for each of us insofar as this world is concerned. Life is an appointment that (1) has God's divine purpose, and (2) requires our accountability:

> *"It is appointed unto man to live and die but once — after this comes his evaluation before God"* (Paraphrase author, Hebrews 9:28).

Contrary to the confused ideas of a few sincere souls, Jesus' words, "You must be born again," do not have anything whatsoever to do with another birth beyond this lifetime. Being "born again" is clearly explained by Jesus Himself. He clarified new birth as an internal renewal, and He specified our need to experience it in *this* lifetime — to do so by welcoming Him into our life as Savior and Lord (John 3:1-12).

Another realm of error distills from the poetic notion that, while not a recycled personality having lived life before, each baby had existence prior to the womb. This scenario somehow envisions God as a Heavenly Father doling out angel-spirits across the earth; installing them in baby-bodies either before or at birth. This unscriptural and insensitive idea is at the root of the frequently parroted statement, so sincerely spoken at the funerals of young children, that God somehow "knew better" and that He *"took back"* the life He had earlier given from heaven.

However well-intended the thought, God didn't and doesn't "take babies because He needs them in heaven." The pain and problem of death exists on this planet because humanity has breached its trust with the treasure of life. And the Bible doesn't say anything at all about God making independent decisions about the placement of each life into each body. Let's see what it *does* say.

Genesis 2 elaborates what Chapter 1 introduces: God, having created man, told him to be fruitful and multiply. Now the Word of God relates how man's possibilities and capabilities for this "multiplying" were given by his Creator. They are summarized in these words:

> *"And the Lord God formed man of the dust of the ground and breathed into his nostrils the breath of life, and man became a living being"* (Genesis 2:7).

Literally, the Hebrew text reads that God, in creating the father and mother of the race, placed *in them* the capacity to beget life: "He breathed into them *chayeem* — the breath of *lives*." Notice closely the plural — God gave mankind the gift of *lives*. The concept transcends the obvious Creator-gift of life for each one to *experience*, and reaches further to the gift of *lives* placed

16

within each one's capacity to *beget.*

That one phrase — that God breathed into man *lives* — clearly reveals how God has endowed mankind with *both* (1) the *capacity* to beget life and (2) the *responsibility* to do so. The ramifications of this fact are profound.

First, this ability has been placed at man's discretion. Each time the conception of a child occurs, God does *not* have to take separate action to infuse the fertilized ovum with life. Life is simply *inherently present* — instantly, spontaneously, always *there,* because God delegated "lives" to man for propagation. The awesome ability to reproduce eternal *souls* as well as physical *bodies* has been given to mankind.

Second, until that union of sperm and egg occurs, *man* is the steward of that life-begetting potential. No given number of off-spring is mandated by God. God never indicates a requirement as to quantity, but only that there be a will to say yes — that we *will* have children, in obedience to His command, "Be fruitful . . . multiply" (Genesis 1:28).

Contrary to some sincere people's thinking, the Bible does *not* say birth control is wrong. God has given man the responsibility of governing the *multiplication* of life. While He *has* commanded him to *beget* children, He has *not* mandated an interminable abandonment to chance, or required a given number of offspring; (or assigned us to *in*numerable ones!).

What the Bible *does* say, however, is that children are a blessing and should be *sought* (Ps. 127:3; Ps. 147:13; Is. 8:18). The Word of God employs the loveliest terminology in describing the joy of childbirth, the meaningfulness of parenthood and the desirability of a family. But the Bible further implies that since life begins at conception, the willful extinguishing of that life is *not* an acceptable method of birth control. According to the Word the frequency of conception *can* be controlled, but life once conceived cannot be taken at human will. In short, (1) *man is not* to completely avoid begetting children; (2) nor is he to abort those who have been conceived.

So, we see from the very establishing of the creative order:

- God has placed life immediately within man's capacity to reproduce;
- He has called him to exercise that life-begetting capacity; and
- He clearly expects that once life is conceived, its preciousness be honored.

We do not need to go to the laboratory to see if life begins at conception, nor are we at the mercy of volatile emotions on the subject. Rather the cool, crisp words of God's timeless truth show us created man, who from his beginning has possessed the God-given ability to beget another being created like himself. This kind of life is in the loins of *both* the man and the woman when each contributes his share toward the multiplication process, and in the instant those cells conjoin, another life begins.

" . . . God obviously
anticipated our inquiry
centuries ahead of time."

Chapter 2

When Does
Significance Begin?

Not only does the Bible establish the fact of the prenatal existence of the human being — that is, that there is human life as God views human life *before* birth — it further teaches the worth, importance and spiritual viability of each one. David observed how true this is in praising God for how He takes note of and protects the fetus.

> *"For You (Lord) have formed my inward parts; You have covered me in my mother's womb"* (Psalm 139:13).

This text makes direct reference to the deepest part of our being — the "inward parts." The Hebrew term *kilyaw* was the figurative expression used in that language to represent the "foundation of being." Just as we refer to the "heart" as the seat of our being or inner person, the Hebrew tongue referred to the kidneys (*kilyaw*). The use in the Scriptures of this expression, referring to a child in the womb, unquestionably establishes biblical support for the idea that a *spiritual* "being," not only a physical one, *does* exist in the womb.

And notice how God's personal attentiveness toward each fetus is so beautifully declared: "You covered me," David announces; that is, "You came to my help." A close scrutiny of the verb chosen by Jewish translators of this passage reveals that the literal statement of the text is that God is *beside* the child — to *help* it and to *keep* it from its earliest beginning (Septuagint: *antilambano*).

I wonder what David was referring to. During his childhood years, had his mother told him stories of her being especially sustained by God's intervening grace during her pregnancy? Might David be saying that he was spared by some providence, or is he simply making a general statement about God's care for the child in the womb? In any case, the inescapable truth is that His personal attention is stated; a concern which Jesus affirmed God feels for each individual many many times more than His very real Creator-care for a mere sparrow! (Matthew 10:31) Psalm 139 gives us a mighty insight: God views life in the womb as (1) real and eternal; and shows us (2) it is desirable and worth protecting.

WHEN IN THE WOMB DOES VALID LIFE BEGIN?

This question has captured the interest of philosophers and scientists over the centuries, as man has sought to define exactly when life actually begins. More recently, debate has centered on the question as to which trimester — that is, which three-month segment of the nine months of pregnancy — life may in fact become "human."

It seems that God anticipated this specific question ages ago, for in the Bible we have a case in which the most precise evidence is given, showing us that *viable, significant* life in the womb specifically exists during *all* of the first three months; i.e., that *from conception* FULLY MEANINGFUL LIFE is present.

Of course, the biologist has shown the poignant physiological evidences of life in the first three months: The third week, the lobes of the brain are distinguishable; the fourth week, the head and face are recognizable and the heart starts to beat; during weeks five and six, the eyes are identifiable and legs are putting on flesh and muscle; in the eighth week the embryo moves to the fetal stage and the following weeks, sex can be identified; the baby can begin to turn its head, squint, frown, make a fist and even get the hiccups: all of this is *before* the end of the first three months in the womb! (Source — LIFE Magazine reprint, copyright 1965, 1979.)

But as touching as these biological signs of humanity are in the *physical* formation of the babe-in-the-womb, look with me at the pointed evidence the Bible gives of the *personal, spiritual* viability of that child. An unmistakable statement is present here, as God has placed at the heart of His Word a story which reveals the fact of a baby's real, personal meaning-filled existence during the first three months following conception. It's the story that is among the best known of all in the world. Although given to tell us of the gift of our Redeemer, hidden within this story is a precious fact concerning the Creator's basic gift of life itself.

Mary, the young woman of Nazareth, has received an angelic visitation announcing her role as the mother of the Messiah. We pick up the story in Luke, Chapter 1, verse 39.

"Now Mary arose in those days and went into the hill country with haste, to a city of Judah, and entered the house of Zacharias and greeted Elizabeth. And it happened, when Elizabeth heard the greeting of Mary, that the babe leaped in her womb; and Elizabeth was filled with the Holy Spirit. Then she spoke out with a loud voice and said, 'Blessed are you among women, and blessed is the fruit of your womb! But why is this granted to me, that the mother of my Lord should come to me?'" (Luke 1:39-43)

The words of Mary's cousin Elizabeth are astonishingly relevant to the philosophical inquiry of this twentieth century. The precision of the text seems crafted by the Holy Spirit twenty centuries in advance: we are, within the span of thirty verses in Luke's Gospel (v. 26-56), explicitly told:

1. A child has been conceived in Mary's womb;
2. It is spoken of as present, as alive, and as "the Lord" *at that moment* — no less a person for being a fetus; and

3. The *exact chronology* of the event.

In verse 36, the angel told Mary at the same time as *her* conception, that Elizabeth was in her sixth month of pregnancy. In verse 56, we are told Mary stayed with her until the birth of Elizabeth's baby — *"And Mary remained with her about three months."* In other words, when Elizabeth was filled with the Holy Spirit and prophesied upon Mary's arrival — "the child in your womb is the Lord" — Mary was only a matter of a few days into *her* pregnancy.

It's astounding.

It's a prophetic statement cut from the cloth of human experience two millennia ago and unrolled before mankind today. Does the Bible say that life in its truest essence exists from conception?

Absolutely!

Does it specifically answer questions about the first trimester of pregnancy?

Absolutely!

And the most profound revelation to the thoughtful reader and inquirer should be *not* in the fact the question is answered, but in the manifest fact that God obviously anticipated our inquiry centuries ahead of time. The meticulous detail, written without strain to the natural flow of the story, silences the doubts of any who accept the authority of God's Holy Word: Life — personal life, meaningful life, *human* life in its deepest, lasting sense — exists in the womb from conception. We are not only shown the evidences of a real body in formation during the first trimester, but we are given a conclusive statement concerning a real *being* at the same time: a *human* — a lasting, eternal soul — is present from conception.

THE POINT IS PERMANENCE

And what is the point of this exercise in Bible exegesis?

Simply this: To establish a foundation for the *permanent* existence of infants who have been stillborn, miscarried or aborted.

The foundations of hope amid any human dilemma, or in the face of any human disobedience, will always be drawn from God's Word — not from human reasoning or happy-talk philosophizing. And the beginning point of the hope I want to offer in consolation to anyone who has lost a child by one of those three means is in underscoring that your child *still* exists! It not only *was* a real, valid, meaningful person from the instant of its conception, but it has *continued* to be a real, lasting, eternal being since the moment of its death.

- That miscarried child did not disappear as a being simply because a clump of tissue slipped from its grip in the womb.

- That aborted baby did not cease its larger existence simply because a surgical instrument or vacuum scraped or sucked its physical existence into oblivion.

- And to the parent of the stillborn, or to those who have held a dead baby in arms — one who died so shortly after birth, seeming to have flown before it was truly known, caught away by an early flight — I tell you, that child's soul — and the same with the miscarried and aborted — is no less caught up to God's presence as an eternal being than the soul of a ninety-year old man or woman, dying and going to their Maker.

The Word of God — the Creator's "handbook for humanity"—gives us understanding at this initial point of inquiry: What about the relative reality of life with the blastula, the embryo, the fetus, the stillborn? His answer: *It's real.* And therein a biblical point of hope is present, for this means that your lost child is in God's presence, and you will some day meet him or her.

FOR SOMEONE, A DILEMMA

But I can almost hear someone asking, "If the baby I aborted is one I will some day meet, will he — will she — accuse me for disallowing it life as I have been allowed it?"

What a poignant question.

What a potentially haunting specter: to arrive in the afterworld, to stand in the presence of God and to be indicted *not* only by the Almighty Himself, but to be confronted by a being never really known, but in that moment completely recognized. How unimaginable, to have that person rise, pointing to you and say, "That is the one who bore me . . . and the one who denied me life on earth." What a stark, raw, emotion-shattering question! Could such a moment be?

On the grounds of God's Word, the answer is NEVER!

NEVER!

Because any judgment before God's Throne will be declared by Him alone. He will not marshall witnesses against us, for it is solely with Him we have to deal when we give our accounting, and He is the faithful witness of all our lives (Hebrews 4:13; II Corinthians 5:10).

And the fear of recrimination for ANY sin or failure NEVER needs to cloud your soul, because the largest fact in the universe is the fact of God's provision for *all* of our forgiveness:

"For God so loved the world that He gave His only begotten Son, that whoever believes in Him should not perish but have everlasting life." (John 3:16)

And your or my relative undeservedness of such merciful love and great forgiveness is not an obstacle:

"For God commended love to us, in that while we were sinners, Christ died for us." (Romans 5:8)

The happy and holy consequence of Christ's death for our sins is that complete payment has been made and joyous gladness for complete forgiveness is fully available to you and me today.

Let me ask you something — not merely if you've felt shamed, guilty or tainted by your part in the sadness of an abortion. Indeed, that may never have been a failure on your part. But all of us have sinned, and honesty before God brings a sense of condemnation for things now, in your past — or factors very much in your present. Is this so with you? Honestly?

Listen. There's good news today.

God's provisions for our past are not only sufficient, but His promise for our future is incredibly bright! A brilliant light shines from the face of Jesus, not only burning away the darkness of sin-shadows which seek to engulf the soul, but radiating a beam of brightness into the future.

Open your heart to Him — to His love, His hope and His comfort: *"For as many as receive Him, to them He gives the right to become children of God."* If you've never asked forgiveness for past sin, *of any* or *every* kind; or if you've never invited our Savior Jesus Christ to enter your life in healing love and saving power, do it now.

Prayerfully bow and speak your heartcry to Him.

And having done so, in the spirit of peace which His healing truth and love can bring, questions about those little ones who have taken the early flight are answered by a new level of hope, elevated by the fact that your soul has had its greatest need supplied:

A Savior.

"Our investigation of such questions must be more than merely theoretical or theological, and in making the Creator's Handbook our textbook, we have substance, not theory."

Chapter 3

Life to What Degree?

In the light of God's eternal Word, we have established the fact that life does indeed begin at conception; that even before birth a fully significant being has begun its realization of the Creator's purpose for its own self.

In discussing the aborted, miscarried or stillborn, another question rises:

Since the body never reaches completion, as with the miscarried or aborted:

Since it never grows beyond birth, as with the stillborn;

Since those lips never cried, much less spoke intelligibly;

Since that tinyness hardly thought reflectively ... never really made a self-conscious assessment of its own being;

then,

what is the exact nature of that undeveloped "eternal being"?

The popular consensus would be that the child never was, or if it "was" somehow, no longer *is*. The natural deduction of the mind un-enlightened by divine revelation would be that the infant life so sadly wasted either by physical malfunction or decisive human intervention, could never realize a destiny — indeed, probably never had one. But just as ignorance forfeits hope, insight can regain it.

We have already found that each child has, before birth, a divinely ordained endlessness to its being: Humankind once conceived become eternal souls, since their life does not begin with their first breath or their first heartbeat. It begins at once with the initial uniting of the cells contri-buted by the mother and father to the possibility of each child's becoming. From that moment, according to the Bible, a viable being exists; a being which transcends its relative physical dura-bility — be it eight hours within the womb or eighty years beyond it.

This being God's conclusive word on the sub-ject, we may logically ask, "Then what is the eter-nal destiny of the unborn or stillborn child? If the child never knew a life on earth, what becomes of it? What purpose? What intelligence has it? Indeed, it may be eternal, but an eternal 'what'? To what degree does this life exist?"

GROUNDS FOR UNDERSTANDING

Our investigation of such questions must be more than merely theoretical or theological, and in making the Creator's Handbook our textbook, we have substance, not theory. We are not guessing, for God's Word of truth eliminates guess-work. Neither are we theologizing for the sake of academic argument. God didn't give His Word as a text for forming ritual creeds but as a source for answering human need.

Our foremost need is to know God's love and forgiveness, but with this we also need the hope He extends. Only His Word offers the pathway to discovery of His purpose; a functional purpose that brings both meaning to our lives and strength to rise beyond our weaknesses. God has given insights in His Word which can counter our doubts and conquer our fears, bringing lasting hope that our failures or disappointments need not preempt our possibilities.

This is what God's program of redemption is about: The restoration of life and hope. He forgives us to give us a future, and He redeems us to begin a program of restoring all that we have lost, whether through our helplessness, our ignorance or neglect, our failure or sin.

Thus, with direct reference to the subject of the destiny of those little ones who have taken early flight from this world, we have reason for great expectation. Examination of the solid ground of the Scriptures elaborates more of the nature of their being and gives footing for faith in a future beyond our heartaches. To determine exactly what the "early flight" child may be or become beyond the womb, we must answer these questions:

1. Is that being sensitive and responsive as a spiritual entity? Is there evidence that it possesses insight or "intellect" in the

most spiritual sense of the word?

2. If so, is there a positive eternal destiny ensured for these children we never knew? What of heaven? *Where* in heaven? Or, heaven at all?

The Bible is anything but silent about the spiritual nature of these little ones and yet I had never heard any teaching concerning these questions; so little, it seems, has been addressed to these issues. I confess, I would never have begun this quest to probe these passages were it not for two factors.

First, as pastor of a large, growing urban congregation, I was repeatedly encountering believers, newly born again to faith in Jesus Christ, whose past contained the pain of memories related to abortion. They wondered about the life of the one they had extinguished from this planet.

Second, an unusual and very interesting conversation took place. Let me tell you the story.

My wife Anna and I were talking with an older lady one day; a dear saint who had been a part of our congregation. Over the years we had come to know her as both a sensitive and sensible person. She was never given to flights of spiritual fancy; in fact, she would resist any kind of fanaticism, yet in her openness to the Holy Spirit's dealing in her life, she truly did on occasion hear from the Lord. Except for the fact that she was such a balanced, spiritually-minded, scripturally-ordered person, we probably would not have been ready to put much stock in the episode she related. In a nonmystical, very natural and unaffected way, she recounted the following:

"Shortly after my husband and I had our first child, I almost immediately became pregnant again. Because we were so young, because it was during the depression and because neither of us knew Christ or God's Word of promise, we sought and I experienced an abortion. Some years later, after our other children were fully grown, I was at prayer one day — not even thinking of this long-past fact of our lives — when the Holy Spirit said: 'You have never presented that child to the Father.' I was quite taken back, not because I felt shamed or condemned but because, well, first, I hadn't even been thinking about that abortion experience. Second, it would *never* have occurred to me to *ever* make an actual dedication of an aborted child to God.

"Still, the experience being so clear, I spoke with my husband about it, and after prayer and studying the Word of God, we did exactly that — together. We knew we had long since been forgiven for the sin we shared at that time, in our ignorance of God's better way. But now we simply prayed: 'Lord, You are the Father of all spirits. Your Word says so, and we believe You not only gave us an eternal soul whose body we mistreated in our ignorance, but whose being still exists within Your great domain. Knowing nothing more, we humbly come to present this child You gave us — to present it to You. And we do this in Jesus' Name. Amen.'"

Now, that couple did *not* feel that prayer was accomplishing some "salvation-by-proxy" or any such foolish notion. Nor were they presenting a new doctrine or some pattern of behavior they felt should be observed by everyone who shared their particular failure. To the contrary, they simply were responding to something they felt within their own hearts. That act of dedication was not so much for the baby's benefit as for their own, for the experience helped them to a genuine realization of the fact that their baby still exists — something they had not considered as deeply before.

As for me, it was the hearing of that episode that finally prodded me into a diligent study of the Scriptures. As a result, I not only was moved, edified and enlightened by the Word as I pursued this theme for teaching the congregation, but since then I have shared these truths with countless numbers via the media.*

A GLIMPSE FROM JEREMIAH

So now we come to the question of the *spiritual* capacity of the unborn child. Begin with me at the words of the prophet Jeremiah. Although it is clear in the text that Jeremiah is specifically speaking about God's Word to him personally, the Bible is equally clear that God is no respecter of persons. He is as committed to *each* of us as He is to *any* of us, and it is in that understanding our glimpse from Jeremiah becomes a look at God's view of each of us — while we were yet unborn:

> *"Before I formed you in the womb I knew you, and before you were born I consecrated you . . ."* (Jeremiah 1:5a)

The prophet pointedly attests to God's revelation that man's prenatal existence is but part of and linked completely to a postnatal one; in other words, the life of our soul is an eternal, spiritual continuum which begins at conception and continues through and beyond birth. Just as our bodies experience a *temporal* physical continuum which begins in the womb and continues growth and function beyond it for our *earthly* lifetime, so our spirits — the essence of our life — exist from conception and beyond for our *eternal* lifetime.

While notably underscoring the ongoing spiritual viability of the child who never experiences the potential of life outside the womb, this verse yields two giant facts about *every* human: the *first* reveals divine intent, or purpose; the *second* reveals divine input, or provision.

INTENT AND PURPOSE

The words, *"Before I formed you in the womb I knew you,"* do not suggest the preexistence of the personality but they do teach God's pre-awareness of and intent for the child. He is saying for each of us to understand, "None of you is an accident. I have foreknown your conception. I have pre-planned and provided purpose for your life." To personally apply the essence of this concept can be mightily transforming for any of us.

In private counsel I have met so many people whose sense of personal worth was repeatedly demeaned during their childhood by such remarks as, "We never planned on you"; "If we had known what we were doing we would have had fewer children," etc. Such depersonalizing feelings are often accentuated when people discover they were illegitimate offspring or the products of some extra-marital affair. Individuals wonder about worth, despair of destiny, and often succumb to feelings of pointlessness — especially in a society which argues for *chance* as the explanation of man's creation rather than God's *purpose*.

But to all human fear, blindness, sin and misgiving, God speaks from His Word: He was not caught by surprise where *any* of us were concerned! "Before you were formed in the womb, I knew you." Let that deep, deep statement of His primary intent and purpose for every human being seep into *your* soul, and let it be a hallmark of our awareness about each child in the womb. Whatever the frustration, inconvenience, pain or displeasure, there is no being without purpose in the larger providences of God. His purposes may not always harmonize with ours, but in the eternal symphony we will come to recognize better the part played by each creature . . . even when the note played by circumstance seems dissonant.

INPUT AND PROVISION

Jeremiah 1:5 illustrates that God's purpose for people is already in force — in His mind and intent — while they are yet in the womb. "I have appointed you a prophet to the nations," God said of Jeremiah; and in respect to a planned purpose, he is not an exception, he is an example of God's intent. He is a proof case of the fact that no unborn child is without distinct spiritual significance in God's design.

But there is a second feature in this text, for in saying to Jeremiah, "I have appointed you a prophet," God is not merely making an assignment, He is ensuring a sufficiency. He assigns duty but He gives the ability to accomplish it.

The implied message is that inherent in every child is not only the *promise* of God's purpose but the *provision* of God's power to accomplish the performance of that purpose. I feel particularly moved to point that out, because I have known of people tempted to abort a child through their unawareness of the dual truth this verse reveals. They not only haven't realized that God already has a purpose for the child, but they don't know God's promise of provision. Without hope or faith that He will provide for and help them see that child's purpose realized, fear and unbelief take over. I have even known of abortions performed simply because of fears of economic failure in the practical task of parenthood.

But God has a promise for such a person: If you'll let His purpose be realized in the child you may fear having, He'll help you at every point. Ask Him for wisdom, and claim His promises to provide an adequate supply for material or monetary need. Ask and you will receive — and your joy in your children shall be full!

SPIRITUALLY SENSITIVE?

Is the unborn child a viable, real spiritual entity — a creature with God's purpose and power in beginning measure; a being with a sensitivity to the Almighty and His designs?

A classic case in evidence takes us back again to the Gospel of Luke, but this time to consider another baby, John the Baptist, who was yet in his mother Elizabeth's womb. The same passage we read earlier (Luke 1:39-43) amplifies our understanding on yet another point.

With the arrival of Mary, within whom the Messiah Jesus had already been conceived, the child within Elizabeth is prompted to *leap* — literally to jump in response to the present reality that was in the Person of the yet unborn Christ. This is incredibly significant since, of John, an angel had prophesied to his father Zacharias, "He — i.e., John the Baptist — shall go before Him in the power of the Spirit (i.e., before Messiah to announce His presence)." Amazingly — in fact it's almost humorous — the baby seems to be doing precisely that! What John would be doing with intelligent speech and by reason of spiritual cognizance thirty years later beside the Jordan River, he first does as an unborn child!!

This is more than an interesting coincidence: The baby didn't just "happen" to jump. Rather Elizabeth's own testimony attributes her certainty of God's witness to the occasion as being directly related to the baby's leaping within her. Man may call it superstition and we might be tempted to call it coincidental, but the Bible says it was the Holy Spirit at work.

Let no one say the unborn are without spiritual sensitivity or purpose. Intelligence may not have flowered as yet nor speech have been acquired, but a purpose has already been plotted by the Creator. The small human mass within the womb is already tuned to the Spirit of his or her Maker.

In Dr. Thomas Verney's book, "The Secret Life Of The Unborn Child," he notes the difference in the fetus' response, even as early as 4½ months, if either iodine or sugar is injected into the amniotic fluid of the womb. The child reacts disagreeably to the taste of iodine, but drinks at twice the normal rate of consumption if sugar is present. Verney goes on to say that unborn children react to the emotional charges they receive from the mother, noting that if the mother is really looking forward to a pregnancy, "it has an incredible, positive effect" on the baby.

We are unhesitant to acknowledge that the evidence is in as far as the natural realm is concerned. Let us be neither surprised to discover nor hesitant to acknowledge that the Bible tells us an unborn child is at least equally responsive and sensitive to the spiritual realm as well.

Chapter 3, Notes

---

* This teaching was first presented under the title "Short-Circuited Into Eternity" and is available on Cassette #1335 from SoundWord Tapes, c/o Living Way Ministries, 14300 Sherman Way, Van Nuys, CA, USA, 91405.

> "Man without
> a Savior
> is an eternally
> perishable being."

Chapter 4

Destiny in the Afterworld

We've established that the prenatal child is an eternal being capable of spiritual response. Now we ask, if it dies before or shortly after birth, what is its destiny in the afterworld?

At once we open the question of options in the hereafter. Human philosophy suggests multiplied possibilities. God advises there are only two. Man's reasonings offer everything from oblivion to euphoria; from nothingness to anythingness; from extinction like a worm dried on the pavement to an indeterminate number of incarnations as a being moves from one life to another. But God says once concluded on earth, human life proceeds to either heaven or hell.

No limbo.

No nirvana.

No purgatory.

No reincarnation.

No oblivion.

God's Word describes either (1) a destiny *within* His will and desire, or (2) a destiny resulting from *opposing* His will and desire. That these are the only options — eternal gain or eternal loss — is the only fact that gives credence to the extreme measure God's love required to insure the possibility that each person can receive the promise of heaven.

> *"God so loved the world that He gave His only Son, that whoever believes in Him need not perish, but have eternal life"* (John 3:16).

Man without a Savior is an eternally perishable being. That "perishing" is *not* nothingness, but the endless suffering of a created soul separated from its Creator by its own choice and sin.

The Apostle Paul elaborates the depth of this fact, accentuating again how the passion of Jesus Christ, who admittedly came and died essentially to rescue a truly lost humanity, verifies the reality and awfulness of the lostness of mankind.

> *"For the love of Christ constrains us, because we judge thus: that if One died for all, than all died, and He died for all, that those who live should live no longer for themselves, but for Him who died for them and rose again"* (II Cor. 5:14, 15).

The entire motive in Jesus Christ's coming was the love of our Creator who refuses to allow any of us — His own creation — to perish, without the availability of a way back from sin's self-initiated exile. His goal is to bring us back into the present fulfillment and the eternal joy God created us to know.

The fact of limited options in the afterworld being established in God's Word, what does He reveal concerning the disposition of the unborn or stillborn at their death?

TO HEAVEN, OR . . . ?

Our hearts dictate "Heaven, of course!" And as true as that may well be, our answer must derive from greater authority than the convictions of our emotions. Doubtless we would all argue for their instantly being ushered into the Creator's heaven-home forever. And that answer *is* right, but we need grounds superior to our own human sense of justice.

Man's perceptions of justice vary, depending often on his limited viewpoint and are often flavored by presuppositions and prejudice. We need an authoritative statement from the Judge of the universe. What will He say?

With regard to these little ones, as with every human being coming before His presence at their passing, we can rest assured: *God is just.* He does not need any prompting from our emotional proposals. Our insistence that "surely" or "of course" those unborn are "saved" is unnecessary here. God knows the spirit of the rebellious, and that cosmic cul-de-sac called Hell is only a self-imposed place of endless abandonment by people who reject Him. Thus, unsurprisingly, His Word *is* clear concerning these sinless little ones: Their early departure from their short life here takes them immediately into His presence. And our hope can rest in that knowledge on the rock of His Word, not merely on our feelings.

GOD'S WORD ON DEAD INFANTS

A. Jesus' Words.

It is with great tenderness that Jesus speaks of the innocence of little children: *"Their angels*

do always behold the face of My Father" (Matt.
18:10). His meaning is clearly that, notwithstanding every child's inherent potential for sinning, small children, yet in their innocence, still enjoy an uninterrupted discourse with the heart of God. At what age this is broken cannot be calendared, for it would vary with each person. Still, one thing is clear: An unborn or stillborn child hasn't transgressed that union.

B. David's Song.

In the Old Testament David spoke of his departed son who died but days after birth: *"I shall go to him . . ."* (II Samuel 12:23). This statement is broadened in its significance when we note that it was spoken by the same lips which sang, *"and I shall dwell in the house of the Lord forever"* (Psalm 23:6). The place of eternal dwelling for the child now gone was known to be the same place anticipated by the believer who has received God's promise and redemption.

C. Abraham's Cry.

When God told Abraham He was going to destroy Sodom and Gomorrah, Abraham asked, *"Will You indeed sweep away the righteous with the wicked?"* He seems to be appealing to God in the interest of the innocent. Then, he apparently remembers that He doesn't need to goad God to do good, and at once he answers his own question, *"Far be it from You to do such a thing, to slay the righteous with the wicked, so that the righteous and the wicked are treated alike. Far be it from You. Shall not the Judge of all the earth deal justly?"* (Genesis 18:23-25).

Yes! A thousand times, "Yes!" The Judge of the Earth *can* be counted on *always*. He will do justice. He will do right. Always!

As with Abraham and with us and our children, God is fair on *heaven's* terms, not merely earth's. And in those eternal, abiding policies, the message of the Word teaches that the stillborn, miscarried and the aborted do indeed pass into the presence of God.

WHAT ABOUT THE UNSAVED?

"But what if the parents are not believers?" Doesn't the Bible say something about the child then being outside God's grace as I have described?

This question is probably raised on the basis of a misunderstanding of I Corinthians 7:14: *"For the unbelieving husband is sanctified through his wife, and the unbelieving wife is sanctified through her believing husband; for otherwise your children are unclean, but now they are holy."*

But this passage has nothing to do with the spiritual viability of the offspring of a spiritually mixed marriage, nor to do with the children of a couple neither of whom are saved.

In this text, the Apostle Paul is addressing a moral question. The Corinthians were wondering about the legitimacy of children born to a couple where only one confessed Christ as Savior. Was their relationship impure, unholy — and thereby their children illegal or unsanctified in God's eyes? Paul's answer is swift and direct: "No, the children are in no way reduced in God's eyes"; they are declared socially and legally acceptable in God's sight. But in saying this, the Bible neither declares nor implies that parents determine the eternal destiny of their children. Believing couples do not automatically produce believing children, and conversely, nonbelieving parents do not doom their children to eternal loss.

Salvation is always an individual choice. Parental influence during the child's lifetime does contribute very positively or negatively, but it cannot control it. As to the destiny of the unborn, since the children have made no moral choices, they have remained innocent. Thereby God's perfect justice receives them into His presence, irrespective of the spiritual condition of the parents — and without consideration of what the circumstance of the child's conception may have been.

In listening to all of this . . .

Why does so much confusion, misunderstanding and condemnation surround us? Why do so many people wonder about purpose in their lives? Why does fear win over faith, and why are babies snuffed out in the womb like candles in the wind? Why does guilt successfully maintain its grip over so many in spite of the fact that God's forgiveness is so freely offered? Why does smallness of spirit compel believers to sit in judgment on human failure rather than to minister comfort and hope?

The answers to these questions are summarily handled, answered in their entirety in one direct statement which Jesus made:

"The thief comes to steal, to kill and to destroy." (John 10:10)

According to Christ, precisely what we are addressing is the work of the devil; a satanic *theft*

48

of joy, a demonic *killing* of hope and a hellish *destruction* of lives. But the solution to mastery over our arch-opponent's workings is in Jesus' ensuing words:

"But I am come that they might have life, and that they might have it more abundantly" (John 10:10).

Here is truth: the child of early flight — the stillborn, the miscarried, the aborted — is not a "nothing" that has gone nowhere.

- He or she is not a glob of cells washed down a drain, or a mass of bones and tissue thrown into a plastic bag.

- That stillborn child is not a stiffened corpse laid in a small coffin.

Rather, each of those little ones are present with the Father. They have identity, individuality and deserve to be known for what they are — eternal beings. They still have a divine purpose which, though it may transcend our understanding for the moment, we shall perceive clearly when the day dawns that we no longer see as through a glass, darkly, but then face to face (I Cor. 13:12).

If comfort is what you need, I want to touch your hand. I want to pour the oil of hope into your heart if the flame has flickered and needs fuel to brighten tomorrow.

My friend, the truth can set you free — and the truth with which we deal is the Holy Spirit's key to your release. Whatever your heart calls for, whether remote to the immediate subject or directly in the center of it, let's call to Jesus Himself. He is the Truth incarnate and readily present. Invite His working into every facet of your present moment with your heartfelt prayer:

Come, Lord Jesus.

49

"Now there are heavenly
bodies and there are
earthly bodies and the
glory of each is
different from the other."

(I Corinthians 15:40, paraphrase)

Chapter 5

In Heaven As A Person

To summarize, we have examined these truths from the Bible:

1. From conception, the life begun not only is truly human, but it is thereby truly an endless being. An eternal soul exists.

2. Each unborn being has viable spiritual sensitivity. Although intellect and speech as we know it may not have begun, sensitivity, spiritual potential and distinctly human capacities are present.

3. God places inestimable value on and has planned purpose for every human life, so much so that He gave His Son to recover from eternal loss all who will receive His redemption.

4. The unborn or stillborn at death *does* immediately pass into the presence of God — i.e., goes to heaven.

The sum of these statements is that the aborted, miscarried or stillborn child *exists*, *it is* with God as an eternal soul, and it is capable of spiritual, sensitive communication. But still another question reasonably comes to mind.

If the unborn child having died does actually go to heaven, in what form does it appear there? Since the child never developed beyond an embryo or fetus how would it appear in heaven? And even a stillborn child, though usually physically complete, generally has little distinct physical indentification. How does it look in eternity?

Are such questions important?

I think so.

I think so, because we are *all* creatures destined for eternity. Incorporated in God's presence in that eternal city will be all those beings who left before birth, as well as all of us who survived for a lifespan beyond it. We will meet one another there, and we will meet those infants. Once the horizons of that perspective open up, they may garner for each of us a host of biblically-based values.

1. Meaning comes to the miscarrying mother: "I may not have been able to receive my child *now*, but my pregnancy was not a waste of time."

2. Hope comes to the parents of the stillborn or early flight victims: "We never got to know you . . . but we shall, some day."

3. Comfort and forgiveness may capture the one who chose to abort, upon realizing, "God's grace is not only greater than

my sin, but His power and purpose in *life* extend beyond it and can redeem what I exercised of death."

The point is not to suggest indifference toward the wrong of abortion, but to minister encouragement and comfort to the *other* victim; the parent who found out too late how much they really cared for the child now gone.

Here God's Word shines again as so often it does in the dark night of human pain. Consider what it says about a possible *meeting* with the child which left you before or shortly after birth.

A MEETING SOME DAY

In the Old Testament, a marvelously tender story appears — a factual piece of history which climaxes a case of failure with a hope-filled promise.

You've heard the story.

From the balcony of his home, David sees his neighbor Uriah's wife bathing. Filled with lust, he orders Bathsheba to his room and makes love to her, even while her warrior husband is away at battle, serving the very man who is taking his wife. The sordid details of the story result in Bathsheba's pregnancy, Uriah's murder and David's indictment by Nathan the prophet. "The child shall not live," Nathan declares.

Shortly after its birth, the baby begins to decline — death seems imminent. David seeks God's mercy with repentance, fasting and prayer; refusing food in order to intercede before God in behalf of the child.

When the child dies, David is not embittered, resentful nor any longer mournful. His servants are bewildered by his rising from prayer and his ceased mourning. And there, against that ancient backdrop of human ignorance about God's higher purposes for children who have died, David speaks the word of revelation — the word of God's truth. *"He shall not come again to me, but I shall go to him"* (II Samuel 12:19-23).

Take special note of these words.

They are spoken by a man who sinned. Let us especially see how God-given hope springs in the breast of the very person who is in fact charged with being the *reason* the child didn't survive! But he is also a person who both lamented his failure and repented of it. And now he's speaking with hope: "I shall go to him."

David lived a long life following this episode, but here he is saying: "The day will come when I will meet that child, will greet that child, and I will some day forever be with that child."

That's in the Bible, friend. This isn't myth, fable, legend or a selection of poetic thoughts for the sorrowful. This is truth to set us free. Here we are specifically freed to expect to meet children in heaven, to recognize them and to be with them.

HOW SHALL THEY APPEAR?

"But, Jack," I can almost hear somebody say, "What about the miscarried and aborted babies? How do they appear? How could I know or recognize them? In what form are these?"

Thankfully, the Word of God provides us with enough information that those are answerable questions too. While David was referring to a baby who died a few days after it was born, we can authoritatively answer concerning even a miscarried embryo which may have been only weeks along the way toward birth.

From I Corinthians 15:40 we gain our first footing:

"Now there are heavenly bodies and there are earthly bodies, and the glory of each is different from the other" (paraphrase).

The Bible makes two things clear; people who have departed earth's order of things are not wispy spooks, blowing in the wind. Satanic deceptions employ such ghostly projections and are practiced by occultists who conjure up horrifying demonic presences that delude, bind and purvey fear. But the few times we see people in the Bible who, to use the scriptural term, are in their "heavenly bodies," they are identifiable.

When the disciples on the Mount of Transfiguration saw Jesus talking with Moses and Elijah, they recognized human beings and intuitively knew who they were. They didn't witness double exposure-type pictures, nor were they struck dumb or horrified by ectoplasmic mirages. They saw *people* who had died. The Bible in fact distinctly mentions Moses' burial; and Elijah's experience, though unusual, did not preempt actual physical death. Of course, the disciples had never before seen Elijah and Moses and yet they knew immediately who they were.

"But how will I recognize someone who never had a body?"

This is more than a reasonable question. It is a difficult one. After all, if the miscarried or aborted child was not even completely formed at the time of its passing, what is there to meet . . . to greet?

GOD'S RECORD OF YOUR APPEARANCE

Psalm 139 is an ode to the wonder of God's genius and love in providing us with the incredibly marvelous equipment we call the human body. In verses 15 and 16, the Psalmist writes, *"My frame was not hidden from You, when I was made in secret, and skillfully wrought in the lowest parts of the earth. Your eyes saw my substance, being yet unformed. And in Your book they all were written, the days fashioned for me, when as yet there was none of them."*

Here, thirty centuries ago, is fantastic advance notice of something we have only begun to understand in this century. The writer is saying, "Lord, all my members are written in your book . . . even while they are yet being formed in the womb, you already have a record of what I shall physically become." The New English Bible puts it with this crystal clarity: *"Thou didst see my limbs unformed in the womb and in the book they are all recorded; day by day they were fashioned, not one of them was late in growing"* (Psalm 139:16).

What "book" is that to which the Bible refers? Where is the book that lists the details of each one of our body's personal design and detailed development?

As recently as the 1950's, biologists discovered the secret of DNA; the spiralling double helix within the cellular structure of the human body which holds in coded form the details of every aspect of the physical potential. The remarkable thing is that this "book," so to speak, is within every *cell* — the *whole* blueprint. This means, essentially, that even in the smallest collection of cells formulating the tissue of a miscarried child, the encoded message of its physical development and appearance-to-be are already present. In short, God knows what your baby that wasn't born would look like when it was 12 . . . or when it was 28.

This isn't intended to answer every question, for there are some we can only speculate on at the present. But what we have said is not speculation. We are dealing in certainties when we say:

(1) The child you lost *now* has a human physical form, and is not an airy ghost floating somewhere in space.

(2) You will meet him or her some day, and will simply "know" who they are, for we will be in the era where *"we will know as we are known"* (I Corinthians 13:9-12).

(3) The physical form is as unpredictable to you now as it was before birth, but is very possibly like the body their genetic code would have dictated had they lived.

God's Word is amazing, isn't it!
Just like His grace.

> "All truth is for
> action, not merely
> for meditation."

Chapter 6

Instruments of Healing

The statements on the previous pages are consistent with biblical revelation.

We aren't guessing.

And in the light of all we have discovered, the question naturally should occur: "What should I do about all of this?" All truth is for action, not merely for meditation. Because God reveals His will in His Word to direct us, not merely to inform us, our focus in His Word is designed to assist us to a response that aligns with His will. One certainty is that He wants us all to become instruments of love, His life and His healing, and I want to invite you to take some steps forward along that pathway.

First, obey the Word of God.

The truths we've studied have to do with the removal of the confusion that surrounds the destiny of the unborn. The Word shows their significance, purpose and eternal potential, and holds forth the certainty they shall have physical forms in the world to come. This offers amazing hope to people who, from their limited perspective, believe their suffering and their grief was all for nothing. But the Bible offers the prospect of a new world, a new togetherness, a new dimension of relationship.

Now that you have gained a grasp of these treasured truths, the call of God is that you be sensitive to opportunities to share them. In settings where you can appropriately offer the truth you've learned, you can obey the teaching of God's Word by doing so.

In I Thessalonians 4, the Apostle Paul was teaching the implications of the coming of Christ, to people who were uncertain of these matters; helping them understand the facts of how the dead will be resurrected at His coming. He helped them come to a grasp of how the living and the dead who are prepared through a relationship with God, will be gathered together in one grand and mighty reunion, and it is with this teaching that he told them, *"Comfort one another with these words"* (I Thessalonians 4:15-18). This is explicit action *any* of us can take when the Holy Spirit provides opportunity to talk with people who will be receptive to God's Word. Tender moments open hearts, and you and I can help healing truth to find entrance. People who have either violated their relationship with the child via abortion, or who through miscarriage or stillbirth never had the opportunity to cultivate one, all deserve to know how God's grace and redemptive provision offers a new realm of possibility.

Inherent in our study is a call to Christians to be done with any mission of extending or deepening guilt felt by anyone. It is one thing to stand against abortion; it is another thing to stand by its casualties. Never fail to presume the real possibility that a woman who has aborted hurts as much as one who has miscarried . . . or as much as parents who have lost a child through stillbirth.

Our call is to comfort, to bring hope, to bring healing; and there is nothing like truth to mend the brokenhearted or to heal the wounded soul.

Second, receive the truth as it applies to you.

Talk with the Lord about the child you once had who has taken early flight. Be reconciled in your soul concerning any anger you may feel over being deprived of the child you had hoped for.

That loss wasn't God's fault.

We live in a broken, imperfect world and we are members of a fallen race. The residual fallout of that fall continually appears around us in the form of sickness, sin, natural disaster, tragedy and death. God didn't make things that way, and He didn't make you an object of His anger when you suffered what you did.

Be certain your heart is right toward Him. He welcomes your spilling out your tears, your

61

sorrow or your heartache in His presence. He will comfort you. But if you make Him the focus of your frustration, you not only fail to receive the comfort He can give, but you are wasting emotional energy aiming your anger at the wrong target.

Express your heart of love toward the child if you feel the desire to talk to Father God about that. According to the Word of God, there is no communication between the living and the dead, but you can freely talk with God about anything you feel, or discuss with Him any question your heart wants to ask.

Remember the couple who "presented" the child they had aborted to God, years after the fact of their repentance and new birth? That is not a ritual anyone should feel constrained to perform; it isn't necessary. But what *is* necessary is your feeling open in your expression to God, and that is what occurred when that couple did what they did.

I've known people to *name* children they've lost — not the stillborn, but the miscarried. I don't think I would recommend that today; in fact, the Bible says the Father has a new and special name for us *all* when we finally gather in His presence! But again, where any may have done this, it is simply another example of hearts being healed through their *openly* communicating with the Heavenly Father. Ours is not to establish a new ritual or a set of superstitious activities for those bereaved of children by whatever means. I do, however, want to encourage that you talk with "Abba," that's the Hebrew word for "Daddy"; and the Holy Spirit has specifically come to introduce us to that kind of healing, saving, freeing intimacy with the Living God (Galatians 4:6).

Third, make use of published resources to minister to others.

I have several times been on some of America's widest reaching television talk-shows, and uniformly the same thing has happened when I have discussed this subject. The destiny of the unborn ignites a dramatic response: Phone boards light up at communication centers everywhere. One broadcaster said the day I discussed the hope of our meeting children lost through miscarriage, stillbirth or abortion that the telephone response was *twice* their daily normal response. To give perspective on that response, that broadcast was at that time the largest user in all America of the "800" telephone number, surpassing all commercial corporations in handling massive viewer or consumer response.

The point is obvious: People are looking for a resource not only to comfort but to point the way into tomorrow. Materials such as this booklet and the tape mentioned earlier are a beginning resource, and the Lord can lead you to tools that will help rebuild other lives.

THERE IS ONE OTHER THING.

I want to talk with you about a stance I feel is important for thoughtful, concerned people to take — a stance toward the subject of abortion.

It's possibly as challenging and as important as any step we may take toward becoming true instruments of healing.

In one way or another all of us are people walking through a living graveyard.

Everywhere we go, among everyone we meet every day, there are the walking dead. They are people so radically impacted by death in one way or another that they are not only candidates for *healing* . . . they need a resurrection.

Death has come to them in one or more of a hundred forms. There isn't anyone you'll meet today that hasn't been touched by it:

   . . . the death of relationships,

   . . . the death of dreams,

   . . . the death of a business enterprise,

   . . . the death of a loved one.

These aren't negative observations made by one who views life dismally. I'm simply noting the fact that death is present in many, many ways. And you and I have been prepared to bring a living answer!

God is alive and at work!

That's the towering reality that rises above our planet-wide cemetery. Jesus has conquered the power of death and in rising has come to walk *beside* you by the touch of His life to bring His answers to your grief.

But there's more.

He's also come to work *through* you. He wants to use His grace in you as a vehicle to reach people who have been swallowed up by pointlessness, regret and weariness.

He's present to work beside you as *your* Restorer and to work *through* you as an instrument of restoration to others.

Let Him do both.

"This is My body, broken for you . . ."
(Matthew 26:26)

Chapter 7

The Heartbeat of Love

As we find practical steps to take through our studying the truth of God's Word, let's proceed to another level of need. What can we do to help stanch the flow of lost lives and lost hope resulting from abortion?

There are attitudes to be assessed and actions to take — and the heartbeat of both is in one word: LOVE — love that reaches with life to cast out fear.

A great many people have deep feelings about abortion today; feelings that tug, that anger, that pinch and strangle. But I wish everyone who's ever been concerned about or scarred by abortion could have been there that morning. What happened, right in the middle of a worship service with several thousand people present would, I think, affect anyone's thinking. That morning everyone felt good about *not* having abortions — but no one felt smug, self-righteous or superior for having this feeling.

Here's the story.

I'll call her Tammy, to protect her real identity.

Tammy had recently moved to the big city. She wasn't a girl without sexual values, but neither did her life have a spiritual base. Some months into her new city experience and her new job, Tammy met a nice fellow. They began to date and, not because either were generally promiscuous, but because they simply both were human, and because neither had any personal spiritual experience, strength or guidance to help anything be otherwise, Tammy and her boyfriend had intercourse — and Tammy got pregnant.

He ran.

Yep, her boyfriend was scared.

That might not be a very noble response on his part, but before you go too hard on the boy, remember what we're talking about: Two young people, hardly even adults in some respects, though in their early twenties, without spiritual roots, carried away by emotion and . . . Well, this fellow was anything but ready for a family, so he ran.

But Tammy couldn't run.

The problem was inside of her body. And what was only as yet a small mass of cells multiplying at a phenomenal rate every day, brought terrifying fear to the girl.

She was new to the city . . . new to her work environment . . . newly in love — at least she had thought so. And now she was about to become a new parent — and without a partner.

Tammy wrestled with the plaguing fears. She called her parents, and they immediately and completely rejected her; offering nothing of support, guidance or counsel except, "Don't come home." It was then she decided to check the Yellow Pages for some place she might inquire into an abortion.

The previous edition of those same pages, until the new phone book had come out one month before, was much the same as in most cities of our nation. Dozens of abortion clinics were listed — veiled with names that suggest counsel and consultation, but which usually advise "Abort."

Occasionally (in this book there was one) an alternative point of counsel was available. But even then it was not from a Christian perspective — i.e., not with the patient wisdom and gentle power in the touch the Spirit of God brings to any human need.

But, as I said, a *new* phone book had just been published — and for the first time in more than a dozen years since the Supreme Court's infamous Roe v. Wade decision, which brought on the wholesale practice of abortion in the United States, this phone book had a number to call which offered something different. There was an ad — a picture of one hand reaching for another, with the words — "Touchpoint — Free Pregnancy Testing ... Immediate Results — Referrals offered."

And Tammy called.

What Tammy didn't know is that the number she called reached a phone in an office opened only days before; opened because one church caught a vision and thousands of its members believed in it enough to give the funds needed to launch its fulfillment.

The vision was this:

(1) To provide a point of reference for pregnancy counselling without imposing a spiritual demand on the inquirer; but distinctly discouraging abortion — and providing options.

(2) To trust the Holy Spirit to bless their being available by causing hearts to open to the gentle understanding shown.

(3) That by this means, lives would be touched, women ministered to and babies saved.

And Tammy had called . . . which leads back to the worship service I mentioned taking place that special morning; the special day that Tammy came to church with her baby.

You see, following that phone call, a lot of time, a lot of patience and a gracious, unpressuring influence had been shown and given to her. Tammy immediately recognized a quality of life — of love — she'd never known before. The result is that Tammy decided against abortion, a little while later received Jesus Christ as her Savior, and on this special Sunday had brought her newborn baby girl for dedication to the Lord.

Although there was no baby's daddy or husband present beside her, elders from this congregation stood with their wives beside the young woman, and the pastor briefly told her story — having been given Tammy's permission to do so.

Preparing to take Communion, everyone in the room held in hand the broken bread, over which Jesus spoke saying, *"This is My body, broken for you . . ."* (Matt. 26:26). The pastor spoke about the intent of Christ, that through His brokenness a wholeness be ministered to mankind, and at that point invited Tammy and the baby to come to the platform.

The worshippers, though unused to such an interruption at the Lord's Table, listened with tear-moistened eyes as Tammy's story was related. Then the pastor took the baby in his arms and said: "This is as dramatic a case as I think you'll ever see, in which brokenness is made whole through the love of Jesus. This baby would have been broken in the womb, but it wasn't. Because you prayed, you gave and you loved, Tammy found new possibilities, and here in my arms is wholeness, not brokenness."

It was an incredible morning, and all the more wonderful when, shortly after that service, a phone call to Tammy's parents found a changed attitude on their part. Their hearts had been touched that someone, somewhere had helped their daughter in her personal crisis. Now they wanted to do their part.

Today, Tammy is home having been lovingly welcomed there by her folks who are helping their daughter forward in life — with their little grandchild as well.

You'll pardon me if I seem to relate this in a slightly emotional way, because I was there.

I was the pastor.

Ours was the congregation.

I held that baby in my arms and presented it before Father God in the rite of dedication, and my being moved is not simply because a baby's life was spared. It is because the event itself would never have happened had not something else occurred.

It involved three very large steps in a change of attitude. In relating them to you, I risk being badly misunderstood, but I've decided to run that risk. Too many lives are at stake for smallness on my part to prompt hesitation; or, for that matter smallness on any of our part. Because I think there *is* a smallness in many of us, not produced by a willful stinginess of soul so much as by the fear to love.

Let me describe the starting place I was at, and from which those three steps brought me and those who walked that path with me. Because they brought us to a larger place of service and a greater ministering of Jesus' love, let me detail them.

"For God commended His love toward us in that while we were yet sinners, Christ died for us."

(Romans 5:8)

Chapter 8

Three Steps To Loving

I knew the Word of God and I knew abortion was wrong: I opposed it, prayed for people who practiced it, prayed against its spread in our Nation, and I sometimes got mad when I would see television news reports displaying the militant actions of so called "pro-choice" advocates. But earlier in this book I stated that God had changed my attitude without changing my convictions.

For example, I had never had to deal with the victim of forcible incest or rape — a woman pregnant with a baby produced by an involuntary or violent act. Nor had I ever thought much about the agony of soul in a woman whose child within was known already to be deformed. Nor had I considered the emotional plight of the husband whose wife's own health was imperiled to the point that she would probably bear the child at the expense of her life.

Rape.

Incest.

Known deformity in the womb.

Mother's health.

These were issues I had hardly considered. For my part, I was not ready to concede that abortion was the answer to any of these situations. And I must gently say that I'm still not. But at the same time, I have had to come to the point that I not only can, I simply *must* allow for the price of fear — yes, even selfishness if anyone judges it so — when a person chooses abortion in such situations.

Listen.

Listen, please. I make such allowance *not because* I believe it may necessarily be the right choice, but because fallible human beings make wrong choices. And when they do — in the face of whatever alternative counsel I or others can bring to bear on these situations, I cannot . . . not in the Spirit of Christ — I cannot sit in judgment on them for that.

I, too, am a fallible, sinning human being. I, too, have felt fear which has begotten actions less than worthy or faith-filled. And I, too, was being shaken by the Word of God at the point where my self-righteousness toward abortion had been so conveniently sustained. I was being confronted by the Holy Spirit; being reminded that I was to love like He loves.

"For God commended His love toward us in that while we were yet sinners, Christ died for us." (Romans 5:8)

Of course, I knew that verse before, but I always applied it to the doctrine of salvation, never to the duty of a Christian. In other words, I could see how necessary it was that God loved me *first*, in order to reach me with His love. Even though I was ignorant, rebellious, indifferent, sinful — I rejoiced in His loving me anyway. It was — it IS — the truth of the Word. His love is unconditional.

But I'd never had it settle upon my soul that He was calling me to love people like He does. My evangelical orthodoxy required me to insist that I had to resist sin in others wherever I found it. That is, until I thought through the way Christ overcame sin. The way He overcame sin was in surrendering Himself to love — to stand forgivingly before it until *love* overcame it.

Now I was being forced to confront this fact: God wanted me to love people who had abortions, whether I agreed or not. And He wanted me to do it without the usual verbal appendage, "Okay, I'll love them, but I still hate their sin."

I think we may too easily employ that ruse to satisfy our emotional outrage, and when we do, the hatred too often spills over and poisons our best efforts at serving the lost. Can you imagine Jesus on the Cross saying, "Father, forgive them, they don't know what they're doing . . . and I hate it. I can't say how *much* I hate it, but I'll still love them, though I assure you I hate their sin."

Oh, don't make any mistake, my brother, my sister in Christ. Don't think I'm soft on sin, nor am I arguing that God is.

Never.

The reason Christ *died* for sin is that sin is deadly serious business, and the death-price has to be paid in full, one way or the other. When we take matters into our own hands, death prevails. But when we trust what His almighty power has accomplished in *His* dying, life can win!

I was beginning to realize that my attitude was not a necessary part of insuring that payment for sin. God didn't need me to be mad at sin — to hate it — in order to assure it was fully compensated for. He had only commissioned me to be a reconciler — to help people be reconciled to Him by reaching with His love, understanding and tenderness. When I came to terms with the fact that a lot of people aborting children were no less or no more sinful than I was, I found I was far more ready to understand the fears, the emotion and the torment when a woman faced a pregnancy she feared or didn't want. I *wasn't* any more ready to agree she should terminate it, but I *was* more ready to accept the person who made that decision. Then, and secondly, I was now ready to do something about it.

DISCERNING WHAT TO DO

And something does need to be done.

The painful matter of abortion cannot interminably go on being condemned by the indignant while it is promoted by its proponents. The issue isn't only that life's possibilities are being removed from the millions affected, it has to do with attitudes toward the *control* of life; life as it concerns *all* of us — the billions on this planet right now.

Thoughtful analysts of the moral question concerning abortion and who propose that "on demand" privilege be outlawed, are not simplistically pontificating a pro-life cause. They are forcing us to look at the drift which is set in motion once a society accepts the privilege of terminating *any* human life *at* will *and* with impunity.

Where does the process stop?

If life is disallowed in the womb on the front end of its span, what is to stop the eventual evolving of a social policy which may *at* will, *any time and* with impunity, stop it on the other end? If we can legally take a baby's life in the womb, will the next step be taking grandpa's life when he's old; exterminating him as a willful act simply because he's more an inconvenience than a contribution to the community? ("After all, he isn't doing well anyway.")

Euthanasia.

"Mercy killing," they call it.

When suffering intensifies, and the agony of the family looking on is only exceeded by the agony of a loved one in the throes of death while violent disease and indescribable torturous pain rack an aging body, what then?

Who should play God?

That question probes our social consciousness, and people who think abortion is but a single issue, must look into the extended ramifications of its acceptance.

Further, none of this even begins to inquire into the implications of genetic engineering and alternative approaches to conception and child-bearing. No one can forecast the long-range effect of present research and activity in genetic manipulation, recombinant DNA, extra-uterine conception, surrogate motherhood, sperm banks and the experimentation in cloning.

I'm not ready to prophesy the birth of a troop of Frankenstein monsters, but neither can I retire to an ostrich-like stance of passivity, doing nothing about the present trends while pretending they are only passing fads. Man is dabbling in the *control* of life, not merely its reproduction, and there is no scriptural indication that his assignment to subdue the earth and replenish it includes everything he's into right now.

I'm certainly not resistant to the scientific research that has often blessed mankind with benevolent results. But I don't think we can neglect the fact that there are some real negative implications in much of what is happening. Social ethics are spiritual issues, and they are being impacted dramatically by applied biological research.

WHAT IS OUR SPIRITUAL MISSION?

I recently appealed to our congregation to do something to indicate our interest in the life of the unborn child. I wasn't proposing a march on city hall; I didn't offer placards or design a sit-in at a clinic. And I certainly DID make clear my revulsion at the hideous actions of people who bomb clinics in that insane expression of protest. But I further said, "We can't do *nothing.*"

Following that Sunday, I received a letter from a man who I think expresses what some Christians suppose to be a spiritual response: "I don't think the Church . . ." he said, " . . . I don't think the Church should be involved in political issues."

I could hardly believe my eyes: "A political issue?!"

We were talking about *LIFE.*

We were talking about morality.

We were talking about loving people who are afraid to accept the life conceived within them, and trying to lovingly serve them amid those fears.

However well-intended or however supposedly spiritual his motivation, this man reflected the fact that in all of us there is the temptation to find some escape from responsibility for action. I know I would rather leave it all alone; the subject bothers me. But I had to listen to Proverbs 31:8, 9.

"Open your mouth for the speechless, in the cause of all who are appointed to die. Open your mouth, judge righteously, and plead the cause of the poor and needy."

I had (1) faced the facts of my self-righteousness, (2) broadened my perspective on what was happening in some people facing tough situations, and (3) now had taken a hard look at social and moral questions facing us today. But with the third step, what could I do?

Well, I'm not a very political, protest-type person. In fact, I have difficulty with the idea of

"The Church" marching in any arena other than on its knees. I'm sure my feelings wouldn't seem tough enough to satisfy a lot of good Christians, while others would doubtless assess my position as being "too hard."

But I did arrive at a point of action that somehow strikes me as one balanced between judgment and mercy. It involves

   (1) ministering *personally* in the spirit and the truth I've presented in this booklet; and,

   (2) ministering *publicly* by affording people in our society with a living option, through providing the type of resource that resulted in the rescue of Tammy's baby.

The addendum which follows may be utilized as you, or any church leader you have touch with, may wish to pursue. For me it accomplished the third step in loving. I hope it might help you do the same.

AND CONCLUDING . . .

There *is* a turnaround taking place in the thought and actions of many today. I know, because of a massive surge of God's grace which helped me "turn" — to rethink the problems of just one arena of pain tormenting people, like you and me.

I hope this chronicle of my journey, my self-discovery and the ensuing truth-discoveries in God's Word, make a full circle possible. May you know Christ's healing and fullness, and may you become an imparter of His life.

With a heart full of His love and forgiveness, let us each be instant to obey and constant in doing what the angel commended long ago: *"Go . . . and speak to the people all the words of this life"* (Acts 5:20).

Addendum

I have asked my friend, Pastor Geoff Thompson, who developed and launched our church's Crisis Pregnancy Center, to write a few words of practical guidance for any group of believers who are looking for an effective, confrontive, loving and serving answer to the social crisis of "abortion on demand."

But, intercessory prayer is the master key to any transformation in individuals or societies. Geoff has given this information with the understanding that prayer, prayer, and more prayer must precede and accompany any effort. All that we do in seeking to reach, touch and change our world is " 'Not by might nor by power but by My Spirit' says the Lord of hosts" (Zech. 4:6).

*   *   *   *   *

Franky Shaeffer has said that every Christian should picket an abortion clinic. I understand his statement and his sentiments. In 1941, the German people allowed millions of Jews to be hauled off because in the late 1930's, they allowed the Jews to be called "Untermenschen" or "less than people." For *us* to do nothing against the wholesale slaughter of the innocent would be unthinkable.

But picketing isn't the only way.

Sidewalk counselling — approaching women before they enter an abortion clinic and lovingly informing them about other choices — is often successful in changing a woman's mind. Forming a "speakers bureau" to address local high schools and colleges brings the message of life and hope to hundreds.

But one of the best ways to touch mothers, fathers and the as-yet-unborn babies is through a Crisis Pregnancy Center.

Every abortion takes a number of victims. The woman is often confused, pressured, and deceived, frequently facing lasting physical and psychological consequences. In Isaiah 49:15, God asks "can a mother forget her sucking child, that she should have no compassion on the son of her womb?" A woman cannot abort her unborn child without suffering the consequences. A Crisis Pregnancy Center can focus on the woman and her needs, and offer her acceptance, compassion and accurate information about abortion and the alternatives.

The Center can also minister to the father, who may have all the same emotions as the mother, and extend the love of Christ to him, offering forgiveness as well as practical options and wise counsel that will allow his future to be hopeful, rather than hateful.

Through these extensions of love and guidance, the unborn baby is given a chance at life. God calls His people to rescue those being led away to death; hold back those staggering toward slaughter. (Proverbs 24:11-12). Through care and concern with the parents who *can* communicate, we may be able to save the life of a child, who *can't*.

HOW TO START A CRISIS PREGNANCY CENTER

1. Form a Steering Committee

From its inception, a CPC should be developed under the leadership of several persons who represent a wide range of Bible-believing Christians. Proverbs 15:22 states that "Without counsel purposes are disappointed: but in the multitude of counsellors they are established."

2. Contact The Christian Action Council

Since 1975, when it was begun in the home of Billy Graham, the CAC has become the largest Christian organization of its kind, committed to help ministries begin Crisis Pregnancy Centers. With local chapters or constituents in all 50 states and most provinces in Canada, the CAC will assist the development of, and training for a viable CPC. (701 Broadstreet, Suite 405, Falls Church, VA 22046; 703-237-2100)

3. Complete a Community Survey

Using the resources of the CAC, and the manpower of the Steering Committee, take a survey of your community. This information will help to identify the need for a CPC and pinpoint the public and private facilities that are already available.

4. Incorporate and Elect a Board of Directors

Under a nonprofit heading, funds can be raised for the ministry, and the limit of liability and the individuality of the ministry remain separate from any church.

5. Establish Working Committees within the Board

Once the Board of Directors has been established, divide the work into separate committees: Public Relations, Finance, Fundraising, Facility location, Training, Shepherding Homes, Volunteers.

6. Hire a Director

The CPC must COMPETE with a professional quality and attitude of excellence that is equal to or greater than other abortion clinics. For this reason alone, a Director is needed; not only to oversee the operation, but to provide supervision to volunteers. Because this is a spiritual outreach as well as a professional one, the center needs the covering and leadership that a Christian servant can provide.

7. Train Volunteers

The CAC provides hours of intensive training and materials to help your center get off the ground.

Obviously these steps are neither exclusive nor comprehensive, but they do highlight the fact that if God calls you to reach out into your community with the light of hope and the life of Christ, given a vision to do so, you could be just months away from a Crisis Pregnancy Center.

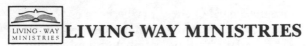

LIVING WAY MINISTRIES

Reaching to touch . . .
Teaching to change

Other Books by Jack Hayford . . .

"The Church On The Way"

In this inspired account of how God taught the people of Van Nuys, Pastor Jack Hayford relates how he and his congregation discovered the pathway to worship; learned how prayer gatherings can be infused with lifegiving power and how genuine faith becomes active in intercession. Here we read about how God "ruined" a man's dream of his own future and gave him a vision of the Glory of the Lord. (1983, Chosen Books).

"Prayer is Invading The Impossible"

Prayer is not the mystical experience of a few special people, but an aggressive act in the face of impossibility — an act that may be performed by anyone who will accept the challenge to learn to pray. Here is a practical "how-to" book that will get you started on the road to effective prayer (1977, Logos International and 1983, Ballantine Books).

"Rebuilding The Real You: God's Pathway to Personal Restoration"

This outstanding study of the book of Nehemiah offers an example of how the Holy Spirit works to restore believers from brokenness. Just as Nehemiah went to Jerusalem with all the provisions he would need to rebuild the walls of the city, so the Holy Spirit comes to you with all you need to be restored in your personality (1986, Regal Books).

Coming Soon From Tyndale House Publishers . . . Jack Hayford's Christian Growth Series:

"NEWBORN: ALIVE IN CHRIST, THE SAVIOR": A practical guide for learning to walk and live in the Family of God, this simple but profound handbook makes a clear statement of exactly what Christ's salvation and one's new birth involve and helps believers discover and understand the meaning and dynamic of water baptism.

"SPIRIT-FILLED: ANOINTED BY CHRIST, THE KING": Practical instruction on the Person and Power of the Spirit, teaching the enablement and resources of spiritual gifts and graces. Encourages the reader to open to the fullness of the Spirit of Christ, and shows how to maintain wisdom and balance in daily spirit-filled living.

"DAYBREAK: WALKING DAILY IN CHRIST'S PRESENCE": Transforms generalized exhortations about "daily devotions" into a workable, nonlegalistic set of specifics as to how the earnest believer can develop a fulfilling devotional prayer life. Not a devotional book; but a practical guide to the individual's own daily spiritual walk with Christ.

"PRAYERPATH": A new call has gone out around the world — a call to believers to unite in concerts of prayer, joining in faith for spiritual breakthrough at a global dimension. The author takes us step by step along the pathway of prayer and shows us what Jesus taught about how to pray and how to live and grow in vital faith.

Also Available From Tyndale House In Spring, 1987 . . .

"THE VISITOR": An intimate look at what it cost the Father to send His only Son to die at Calvary; the depths to which God condescended to bring us salvation. The why's of the necessity of Christ's wounds, His suffering and His death.

To Complement and Supplement Your Reading . . .

AUDIO CASSETTE TAPES . . .

. . . of related teachings by Pastor Hayford are available through the SoundWord Tape Ministry. The following list suggests messages which correlate closely with the theme of "Early Flight."

TITLE	TAPE NUMBER*
"Short-circuited into Eternity"	1335
"Abortion and Adoption"	1521
"Why People Sometimes Die Too Soon"	1451
"Testimony of Triumph"	354

*Please refer to the tape number when ordering.

These and other audio cassette tapes, as well as a complete catalog of messages by Pastor Hayford, are available by writing to:

> **SoundWord Tape Ministry**
> **14480 Sherman Way**
> **Van Nuys, CA 91405-2396**

VIDEOTAPES . . .

. . . may be special-ordered for use in homes, Bible studies, small group meetings and churches. For information and a catalog of current listings, please write to:

> **Living Way Ministries**
> **14300 Sherman Way**
> **Van Nuys, CA 91405-2499**